# CONTENTS

# BOOK DESCRIPTION

This book contains information that you need to know about teething and its home remedies. Signs, symptoms and other problems that your baby may encounter during the teething process are also discussed thoroughly. Through this book, you will learn how to manage teething and deal with other issues associated with it accordingly. This guide will likewise help you make the teething process easy for your babies. Also included in this book are lists of helpful home remedies. These home remedies have been used for many years to treat teething problems.

Here are some of the things that you will learn from this book:

- The teething process and its stages.

- The signs, symptoms and issues associated with teething.

- Various home remedies that are readily available in your medicine cabinet.

- Home remedies that you will find in your pantry and kitchen.

- Old but effective remedies from granny's diary.

# INTRODUCTION

Babies bring joy and happiness in every family. Parents should be aware how to handle their babies, particularly when it comes to proper growth and personal care. Babies show different signs and symptoms as they pass through the different stages of growing up. It is important for parents to know these signs and symptoms particularly in teething process since it requires close attention and proper care. Some babies may experience difficulty during the teething process and there are some who pass the stage without any pain and discomfort. Babies who are experiencing teething problems should be monitored closely.

One of the painful and stressful stages in baby's life is the teething process. It breaks the parent's heart to see their baby in pain and they don't know what to do. The pain and discomfort the babies may experience vary. Some feel more pain while others go to the process without having any pain. There are several remedies that parents can apply to help their babies feel better as they go into the process of teething. Pain-killer medicines, massage therapy, topical gels, herbal medicines and home remedies can help reduce the pain and soreness.

As the babies go through the teething process the pain tends to continue and increase particularly at night time. It's because of the lack of stimulation at night when everybody is asleep and very quiet. This is the reason why your baby cries a lot at night during teething process. The pain may radiate to different parts of his body that will lead to lack of appetite and refusal to take food. The baby may also tend to bite on anything they get in their hands.

Seeing the first tooth is a joy for the parents, but this might be a start of eating disorder, which might lead to various conditions particularly digestive system problems, diarrhea and fever that may cause diaper rash. In order for the parents to manage it accordingly, they need to have enough knowledge about the process and the different home remedies that they can use right away, especially during odd times. These home remedies are readily available in your kitchen cabinets, freezer, medicine cabinets and pantry. With these remedies you can provide immediate relief to your baby's pain and sore gums.

# CHAPTER 01: UNDERSTANDING THE TEETHING PROCESS

Odontiasis is the medical name for teething. It is a process in which the first tooth of a baby appears in a particular sequence by getting through the sensitive gums. Normally the teeth emerge in pairs. It is commonly known as baby teeth or milk teeth or deciduous teeth. Some babies have their teeth in a normal way, and do not experience any teething problems. But, there are some babies who suffer different teething issues, like inflamed gums and soreness, diarrhea, fever and crankiness. For these babies, teething is a painful process as they encounter different problems that are present during teething.

## TIMELINE OF YOUR BABY'S TEETHING PROCESS

As mentioned earlier, one of the hardest parts of the baby's life is the teething process. Most babies start having their teeth at the same age and usually follow a specific order of appearance.

It is a common fact that the baby's milk teeth usually come out in pairs. Majority of the babies experience pain and discomfort when their teeth start to come out of their gums, which makes them finicky and cranky. Parents will feel helpless, particularly the first time parents. To make this situation easier for the parents and for the baby as well, they need to have some knowledge about the physical changes the babies may undergo and how to deal with the situation to help their babies.

Keep in mind that soreness and distress may start even before the teeth appear as babies already have a set of 20 teeth underneath their gums when they were born. You will know when it is time for the teeth to come out when you run your fingers in your baby's gums. There will be notches.

Here are the primary stages of the teething process, which parents should know in order for them to deal with the situation accordingly and provide immediate relief for their baby's teething problems. This will make the babies teething process pain free and easier.

## BETWEEN 5 MONTHS AND 10 MONTHS OLD

Incisors are the four front central teeth. Normally, the first ones that cut through the gums are the two lower central incisors. This stage occurs when a baby is between five months and ten months old. To those who are not aware, teeth growth is hereditary; thus, if your teeth developed early, then there is a higher possibility that your baby will experience teething at the early age as well.

## BETWEEN 6 MONTHS AND 12 MONTHS OLD

The two upper central incisors are the next set of your baby teeth to develop, and normally comes out between six months and twelve months old.

## BETWEEN 9 MONTHS AND 13 MONTHS OLD

The 2 upper lateral incisors on both the left and right side of the center normally appears between nine months and thirteen months old. This will give the baby 4 teeth across the top.

## BETWEEN 10 MONTHS AND 16 MONTHS

During this stage the two lower lateral incisors will appear to the right and left of lower middle incisors. Once these teeth appear, you will be able to see your baby's sweet, toothy smile.

## BETWEEN 12 MONTHS AND 18 MONTHS

Molars are the bigger teeth that normally appear between twelve months and eighteen months. The first molars usually appear at the upper part towards the back of the baby's mouth. The lower molars appear the same time as the upper molars.

## BETWEEN 16 MONTHS AND 22 MONTHS

During this stage the upper canines of your baby appear and fill the spaces between the incisors and the first molars. The lower canines that grow underneath the lower gums will appear the same time as the upper canines.

## BETWEEN 20 MONTHS AND 31 MONTHS

You will now notice the appearance of the two lower second molars on the rear side of the mouth.

## BETWEEN 25 MONTHS AND 33 MONTHS

The final set of teeth of your baby which is the two upper second molars will appear.

## THREE YEARS OLD

Your baby will have a complete set of milk teeth and will display a brilliant smile.

You should keep in mind that the milk teeth of males usually appear late as compared to females. Also the health of the baby is not affected on when and how the teeth will appear.

# WHAT TO EXPECT DURING THE TEETHING PROCESS

One of the common signs that your child is experiencing pain during the teething process is when he cries a lot. Babies handle pain in different ways and as parents, you should know this. Some lucky babies may not experience any pain. But, most babies go through irritable and cranky stages. It's because of sore and swollen gums why some babies are crankier during the teething process as compared to others.

Babies will show signs and symptoms of teething pain a few months before the first pairs of teeth emerge. Normally, these symptoms will disappear once the teeth cut through the gums and come out of it. Babies would normally bite their fingers, hands, toys or anything that is in their hand to relieve the soreness and pressure in their gums. As a result of this pain and discomfort, babies lose their appetite to eat.

Here are some of the common signs and symptoms of teething that your baby might experience during the teething process.

## CRANKINESS AND IRRITABLE

Your baby may become cranky, irritable, crying a lot and uncomfortable as the first pair of teeth come closer to the surface. During this time the gums become increasingly sore and very painful.

## BITING AND GNAWING

Your baby will try to bite and chew anything that they can hold on to. Gnawing helps reduce the inner pressure that the emerging teeth are creating to cut through the gums and temporarily numbs the pain.

## INCREASE PRODUCTION OF SALIVA

If you notice that your baby starts to drool it only means that his teeth are starting to appear. It is normally noticeable when your baby is about 3 to 4 months old. Teething increases drooling and for some babies it could be worse.

## EAR PULLING AND CHEEK RUBBING

Pain due to teething may spread to the ears and cheeks particularly when the molars begin to come out of the gums. This is why babies pull their ears or rub their cheeks. But, also keep in mind that babies also pull their ears when they have anear infection, especially when your baby has fever.

## RASHES AROUND THE CHIN

Your baby may develop rashes around his chin due to an increase in drooling. Use soft cloths or baby napkins to wipe the saliva on his chin and mouth to prevent the chin from having rashes and chapped skin.

## COUGHING

Occasional coughing or gag due to increase saliva could be a sign that your baby is starting to have his first pair of teeth. Cough and flu associated with fever is not a sign or symptom of teething.

## RISE IN BODY TEMPERATURE

Doctors do not consider fever as a symptom of teething. But, there are some parents who find their baby having a mild fever while in the process of teething. Consult your doctor if the fever rises above 101 degrees or if it continues for more than 2 days.

## LOOSE BOWEL MOVEMENT

Most parents noticed that the bowel movements of their babies are a little bit looser. According to the recent studies this is one of the most common symptoms of teething. However, there are some doctors who do not agree with this study. The increase in saliva intake may have caused the loosening of the stool. Check with your doctor if your baby has more than 3 runny bowel movements per day.

## LACK OF SLEEP

As mentioned earlier, pain increases at night due to lack of stimulation at night when everybody is sleeping and the atmosphere gets quiet. This directs the baby's attention to his sore gums, which can result in crying all night as well as staying awake, affecting both the parents and the baby. This is more common when the molars start to cut through the gums.

## COLD-LIKE SYMPTOMS

There are some babies who experience cold-like symptoms during teething like coughing, runny nose, red cheeks and ears, and other cold symptoms. These symptoms are maybe due to too much hand to mouth action to ease the pain. If in case the cold symptoms last for more than 3 days, and do not relieve on their own you can consult with your pediatrician.

Parents should be aware of these signs and symptoms to make sure that what your baby is having are actually signs of teething. Although most parents are sure that the above mentioned are signs and symptoms of teething, visiting your baby's pediatrician is still recommended. There are some symptoms that are also observed in other diseases like fever above 101 degrees and if the symptoms are affecting the baby's health.

# CHAPTER 02: HOME REMEDIES – MEDICINES AND SAFE TEETHING OBJECTS

Teething problems like drooling, lack of appetite, rashes around the chin and cheeks, diarrhea, crying, crankiness, inflamed gums, mild fever, gnawing and ear pulling are normal during teething process. There are some lucky babies who did not experience any of these teething problems. There are things that you can use at home and some safe medicines to help ease the teething problems of your babies. These home remedies are proven to be very effective and safe to use.

Below are some of the medicines and safe teething objects that you can purchase and can be used at home to reduce the pain of your teething baby.

## AMBER TEETHING NECKLACES

One of the most popular home remedies for teething baby these days are amber teething necklaces. Many parents all over the world use these necklaces to reduce the pain their babies are experiencing due to sore gums and teething pain. These amber teething necklaces are made of Baltic amber, according to experts. When the baby wears it, contact with the skin causes it to emit a small amount of oil that contains succinic acid. This is the ingredient responsible for the analgesic effect of the necklace. It also has therapeutic and anti-inflammatory properties that help the teething babies in reducing the pain and discomfort related with teething. All you need to do is to let your baby wear it or get in contact with your baby's skin and it will take effect right away. This will help keep your baby stress-free and remain calm all throughout the teething process. Parents should keep careful watch if you decide to use the necklace as it is a possible choking hazard.

Aside from its healing properties, these necklaces will look good for both boys and girls and even for adults. The amber teething necklaces are available in different lovely warm colors like cherry, honey, cognac, butterscotch and others.

## OVER-THE-COUNTER PAIN RELIEVERS

Over the counter pain relievers can help in reducing the pain and discomfort for 4 hours. One safe medicine for children for pain is liquid acetaminophen, but it is still best to consult your pediatrician as to what is the right medicine for your baby. This will make your baby feel better. Since pain usually worsens at night, taking pain reliever at night will help your baby sleep better. Since it is not recommended to give your babies pain reliever around the clock, it is best to give him the medicine at bedtime especially if other techniques to relieve pain are not working well. Give the right dosage for your baby as advised by your pediatrician.

NOTE: Aspirin is not recommended for teething babies since it may cause Reye syndrome, which is life-threatening.

## FDA APPROVED TEETHING GELS

To help ease the teething pain of your baby, you can use FDA approved teething gels. These teething gels are gentle to your baby's gums and provide comfort and relief from teething pain that will last for thirty to forty minutes. Although the relief does not last longer, they are very helpful in reducing the pain during a tough situation. Some of the popularly used teething gels are Orajel and Anbesol.

## COLD WASHCLOTH

A clean, cold towel or washcloth for your baby to gnaw on can relieve pain and discomfort. Soak a clean cloth in cold drinking water. After wetting the cloth completely, remove it in the water, wring to remove excess water, and then place it in the fridge, until it is cold. When it is cold enough, take it out of the fridge and let your teething baby bite, or gnaw the cold cloth or towel. This will not just relieve swollen gums, but will also make your baby feel better and calm.

## SLIDE YOUR BABY A COLD SPOON

The majority of dental association's recommend using a cold metal spoon in a teething baby's mouth to reduce soreness and pain. To prepare the cold spoon, place the metal spoon in the fridge for several hours and let your baby gnaw it. The pressure of the spoon against his gums will provide relief and will make him feel good and may even put a smile on baby's facc.

## CLEAN MOUTH REGULARLY

Dental specialists suggest cleaning the gums and teeth of your baby regularly. To do this, get a clean wet cloth or gauze and rub the gums to clean the mouth. It will give comfort to your baby and some relief from pain. If in case the teeth have come out already, you can use a soft baby toothbrush to clean the teeth. The babies will be used to cleaning their teeth regularly.

## WRAP ICE IN A TOWEL

Get some ice and wrap it in a new, clean towel and let your baby suck on the towel. This will help reduce the swelling of the gums and lessen the pain that your baby is experiencing. Don't let your teething baby suck on the ice directly or have direct contact on the ice for a longer period of time, as it could harm his gums and cause damage.

## FREEZE BABY BOTTLE NIPPLE

Freezing the baby bottle nipple is another way to help your baby lessen the pain during the teething process. Fill a baby bottle and place in the freezer upside down, to freeze the water at the nipple. Give it to your baby and let him chew on. This is perfect during the most disturbing time of the process. Let your baby gnaw on the frozen nipple, but make sure not to prolong the contact.

# CHAPTER 03: HOME REMEDIES – FRUITS, VEGETABLES AND OTHER FOOD ITEMS

Pain and discomfort are normal in every child's teething process. Since teething is a natural process it is good to treat it also in a natural way. Eating the right fruits and other food items is the most natural approach in managing pain and discomfort during teething. Most of these items are available in your pantry. These fruits and other edible items will help reduce the pain and soreness of the gums of your teething babies.

Here are some of the fruits and food items in your home that you can give for your teething baby.

## YOGURT AND APPLESAUCE

Your babies will love cold yogurt and applesauce because they taste really good and are also gum friendly. These cold food items provide an immediate relief to the distressed and crying, teething baby.

## FROZEN BANANA

Bananas will not just provide relief in teething babies, but also contains vitamins and minerals needed by your growing babies. To prepare, place a peeled banana in the freezer. Give your baby the frozen banana and let him put it on his sore gums. This will provide instant relief from teething pain. It is also the easiest way to encourage your baby to eat something.  Keep in mind that having cold foods on the gums for longer periods of time is not good, so you need to be very careful when giving frozen banana.

Make sure that it will stay in your baby's mouth just long enough to provide relief. Never give something that might choke your baby.

Aside from banana, you can also give frozen pineapple slices. Since it has anti-inflammatory properties and also contains ascorbic acid, letting your baby gnaw on it can provide relief from teething pain.

## OTHER HELPFUL FRUITS

You can also use other fruits, such as apple wedges for your teething baby. Use a clean washcloth to wrap the apple wedges or you can use a mesh teether to hold it. This will not just give your baby an immediate relief from sore gums, but is also the best way to have a fresh fruit juice. Aside from apples, you can also use peaches, watermelon rinds, avocado and pears. These fruits are perfect for your teething babies since they are hard enough to chew on and are easily available. These fruits will not just provide immediate relief but also provide important nutrients.

## CARROTS FOR TEETHING BABIES

Another helpful vegetable for teething babies is carrots. Simply wash it thoroughly and place the carrots in the fridge. Once it is cold enough, peel and let your baby chew it. This vegetable provides your baby not just instant relief from soreness but also the important nutrients your little toddler need. Give your baby a full-sized carrot to gnaw on instead of baby carrots.

If you don't have carrots at home and you have cold celery sticks, you can let your teething baby gnaw it since it is known to be a natural pain killer. You can also try a sliced of peeled ginger root, rub it on the baby's gums. Another vegetable that can provide an immediate relief to your teething baby is a slice of cold cucumber.

## VANILLA EXTRACT

During the teething process , your baby may cry more often and you might have a hard time calming him down. One of the best ways to calm your baby and lessen the discomfort and pain that he is experiencing, is to rub baby's gums with natural vanilla extract. The rubbing will soothe his sore gums. This will not just provide pain relief but it may also help him fall asleep. Vanilla extract is used for toothache since it has a warmed, numbing effect. Simply rub vanilla extract on your baby's sored gums to reduce the soreness. Keep in mind that everything in excess is harmful, so make sure that you use only a small amount of vanilla extract since an excess of it may result to stomach upset.

## TEETHING BISCUIT

You will find a special biscuit made specifically for teething babies. This kind of biscuit is intended to lessen the discomfort your baby is experiencing during the teething stages. The biscuits are hard and unsweetened so your baby can bite on it to lessen pain. As mentioned earlier, biting on something can relieve the inner pressure because of the outer pressure and thus get rid of pain.

## APPLYING COLD BAGEL

Cold bagels, particularly cold whole grain, wheat bagels, are very helpful for teething babies, not only because they are readily available, but also they are hard enough so your baby can gnaw on it. Gnawing cold bagels can provide immediate relief and it can supply the essential nutrients your baby requires. In making cold bagels, simply put an ordinary wheat bagel in the fridge. Through this you can make homemade teething ring. It is used for teething babies to gnaw on as their teeth start to come in. The bagel can ease the pain and discomfort due to teething.

# ARROWROOT COOKIES

Studies prove that arrowroot is very effective in treating upset stomach. But, some parents are using this starchy substance to make cookies for their teething babies. Since cookies made of arrowroot do not break into small pieces easily, it is used as a chewing cooking for teething babies to relieve inner pressure. You can purchase ready to eat arrowroot cookies or you can bake your own cookies.

# CHAPTER 04: HOME REMEDIES – TRADITIONAL BUT EFFECTIVE TEETHING REMEDIES

Traditional home remedies are considered as one of the safest and more effective solution for various problems that your baby may experience during the teething process. These remedies are also known as the "granny remedies" since most of the remedies are handed down by your grandmother. Your grandmother is the most experienced person when it comes to taking care of and raising infants and children. Most of the remedies in this list are natural and do not require medication. Since during your grandmother's time there were no proper medical facilities, pain and discomfort due to teething were managed naturally. Your granny used natural home remedies to treat various medical conditions or illnesses of her baby.

Here are some of the natural remedies your granny has been using for many years now. These teething remedies will reduce the pain and will help you prevent the occurrence of any serious teething problem.

## MASSAGE BABY'S GUMS, CHEEKS AND EARS

One of the symptoms of teething is rubbing of cheeks and pulling of ears. Babies are doing this to relieve the pain and discomfort they feel during teething. So, if your baby is in the teething stage, massaging his gums, cheeks and ears would help lessen his pain. To protect your baby from infection, make sure that you have washed your hands thoroughly before giving a gum massage. To massage the gums, use your clean finger and gently rub the gums. Apply enough pressure on them to help reduce the inner pressure. This will give your baby a great relief from pain and discomfort.

## NATURAL OIL

One way of reducing the teething pain of your baby is by the use of natural oils. This will put him at ease, calm him down, relax and maybe put him to sleep. One of the most common essential oils used for this purpose is the clove oil. Clove oil is effective in alleviating pain. This oil is also used for toothache since it has warming and numbing properties. An adult can place a whole clove against the tooth. This will lessen discomfort and pain long enough to get to your dentist. For your teething baby, simply rub the oil on the sored gums to reduce the soreness. Keep in mind that using too much clove oil can upset your baby's stomach and may irritate his mucous membranes. If your baby is sensitive to clove oil, you can use either German chamomile hydrosol or lavender oil. ( should be diluted according to age) These two are safe for your baby.

## USE FEEDING CUP

If your teething baby is having a hard time eating and drinking his food due to sore gums and sometimes don't want to eat at all, you can use a feeding cup. This will help reduce the discomfort and pain and will improve feeding. Also, various shapes and types of nipples can be used so your baby can bite on it and the outer pressure produced will help relieve the inner pressure.

## GIVE YOUR BABY SOMETHING TO DIVERT HIS ATTENTION

One of the easiest and simplest solutions for teething babies is to divert their attention. It is a fact that pain at night time is worse because they tend to focus on the pain since there are no distractions. One way to divert their attention during the daytime is to play with them using their favorite toys or you take them to the park or mall. Distracting your baby's attention is easy; there is no need for you to exert a lot of effort to divert his attention. You can play peek-a-boo with your baby or give him something colorful to get his attention. Your baby will forget about the pain once his attention gets diverted.

## LET THEM CHEW

Normally a teething baby would try to chew everything that he can get hold on to. It is okay for your baby to chew- just make sure that it is clean and it is big enough so they cannot swallow it. Gnawing or chewing helps relieve the inner pressure, thus reducing pain and discomfort. Experts suggest that you allow your babies to chew on something since it will keep their jaws moving. Make sure that the object is non-toxic and is safe for your babies. Choose objects that are easy for your child to grab on.

## ALWAYS KEEP A SOFT TOWEL HANDY

One of the primary symptoms of teething is drooling. Too much drooling can cause rashes all over your baby's chin and neck. Excess saliva can cause skin irritation, which will result in an uncomfortable and distressing feeling in your baby. To manage this situation, always keep a soft towel handy to wipe dry your baby's chin and mouth. You can also use petroleum jelly or zinc oxide ointment if wiping excess saliva is not enough.

## WOODEN TEETHING RING

In Japan, a wooden kokeshi doll is used for teething babies to gnaw on. This technique for reducing teething pain has been used for centuries and it has a modern alternative. For parents who want natural remedy to alleviate pain, you can try natural wood teething ring with beeswax coating. This ring is safe and environmentally friendly and is a good alternative for plastic toys and teething gels. These wooden teething rings are available online.

The above mentioned home remedies for teething babies have no known side effects. They are easy to use and should be used in moderation. You need to understand that you should use these remedies in moderation. You should use these teething remedies to provide an immediate relief from soreness and pain. Parents are encouraged to first try natural remedies in alleviating pain because it is less harmful before resorting to other medications. These home remedies will keep your baby calm without making you frustrated and annoyed.

# CONCLUSION

Teething is a normal process that infants go through. This is the part of their life where their milk teeth are starting to come in or cut through their gums. The teeth normally erupt in pairs. The pattern on how the teeth appear may vary among babies, but the teething process normally starts at the same age and also the order of appearance of the teeth. There are some lucky babies who go through the process without experiencing any teething problems. Most babies experience teething problems like crankiness, sore and inflamed gums, cheek rubbing and ear pulling, drooling, rashes around the chin, diarrhea and irritability, lack of sleep, coughing and fever.

It is a given fact that teething is a painful and stressful time for both parents and the baby. But with the help of these home remedies, your baby can get an immediate relief from the painful and sore gums. In order to handle the situation effectively, the parents should have enough knowledge concerning the different remedies that they can apply, particularly when their teething baby is very fussy.

Aside from treating your baby's teething problem using different products available in the market today, you can also use some home remedies that are readily available in your refrigerator, pantry, medicine cabinets, kitchen and freezer. These home remedies are very helpful in providing instant relief, particularly when your baby needs it at night time. Also, if you notice these symptoms it is best that you bring your baby to his pediatrician and ask for the best remedy for teething problems especially if your baby has a fever and is affecting your baby's health.

www.ingramcontent.com/pod-product-compliance
Lightning Source LLC
Chambersburg PA
CBHW081142280526
45787CB00007B/3188